MW00445147

5/2 Diet: Intermediate Fasting For Rapid Weight Loss And Health

Celebrity Secrets to Losing Weight

by Salutem

Tunnel

otherwise, by any usage or abuse of any policies, processes, or directions contained within is the solitary and utter responsibility of the recipient reader. Under no circumstances will any legal responsibility or blame be held against the publisher for any reparation, damages, or monetary loss due to the information herein, either directly or indirectly.

Respective authors own all copyrights not held by the publisher.

The information herein is offered for informational purposes solely, and is universal as so. The presentation of the information is without contract or any type of guarantee assurance.

The trademarks that are used are without any consent, and the publication of the trademark is without permission or backing by the trademark owner. All trademarks and brands within this book are for clarifying purposes only and are the owned by the owners themselves, not affiliated with this document.

Preface

In this book you will be provided with detailed information on this very new and interesting diet program, the 5 2 diet. We will teach you exactly how this plan works so that you can maximize your chances of success. The program is based on certain specific principles, and we will explain them to you in detail. You will learn how intermittent fasting can be beneficial to your health but can also contribute to a fast method of weight loss.

Additionally, you will be provided specific meal plans and many examples of foods both to favor and avoid during your weight loss program. You will understand what is happening to your body and how it is in fact possible for you to shed those unwanted extra pounds. You will also discover what else you should be doing while on the program so that you can lose this extra weight for good.

The 5 2 diet, as its name implies, will focus on a program in 2 parts: 2 days of fasting and 5 days eating normal healthy meals. You will be able to choose wisely what you put in your body to maximize the effects of the plan and will soon be very proud and happy with the results. Your commitment to this new healthy lifestyle will pay off faster than other diet programs, and you will soon understand why.

Congratulations again, relax and enjoy taking your first step towards achieving a healthier, skinnier and happier you.

Table of Contents

Introduction

We would like to welcome all beginners to the world of dieting, but we especially want to welcome those individuals who are discovering the 5:2 diet plan for the first time and want to learn in more detail what this wonderful weight loss plan is all about. It is also called the fast diet, and you will soon fully comprehend why.

This diet plan is fast becoming very popular in The United States, the UK, and Europe. So, get ready to be impressed. Actually, many famous individuals already adopted this diet plan. That's right, male and female celebrities, including Beyoncé (singer), Miranda Kerr (model), Ben Affleck (actor), Jennifer Lopez (actress, singer), Jennifer Aniston (actress), Phillip Scofield (showbiz), Dom Joly (comedian), have lost weight using the 5 2 diet. They all mentioned how simple to follow but efficient this diet plan was for them.

Not only do we want you to feel better and lose weight fast, but we also want to teach you to adopt a new permanent lifestyle that could help lead to a much more fulfilling life.

Two days where you restrict yourself, and 5 days where you eat normal healthy and balanced meals, doesn't sound so bad, does it? Most diets ask you to watch what you eat every day, count the calories, or weigh your food 7 days a week. There's no need to do any of that with the 5 2 diet, as it will allow you to choose 2 non-consecutive days a week and practice intermittent fasting.

This book will explain to you how and why you should practice fasting in your life. It will make it easy to understand why it is so efficient and what happens in your body that you can be confident in losing weight as fast as you want when put your mind to it. Discover the other benefits fasting can bring in your life if done correctly and safely. There is no need to be scared or apprehensive, as you will learn what to do and not to do while you are fasting. In this particular case, it does not mean to go completely without something to eat or drink. It simple means that during the chosen 2 days a week you will eat a lot less than the other 5 days. Again, we will assist you in picking the right foods and right quantity to be successful at your weight loss goals.

You will be so pleased that you have adopted this diet plan for the long term. It this is why we will place an emphasis in this book of promoting all the advantages of sticking with this diet for the long term benefits. Unlike other diets where you will are starving and can't wait to get off the strict regimen and go back to your normal habits, this 5 2 diet plan will help you create an easy to follow routine. You will feel better and be more energized.

Finally, since this diet plan has been undertaken by many already, we will be able to provide you with answers to the most commonly asked questions people have had already. So don't worry, as you will not enter this diet plan blindly. You will be very well informed and educated to ensure that this plan is right for you. Additionally, we want to give you all the tools needed to succeed in your mission of weight loss by giving you a plethora of tips that will be useful to you.

Chapter 1
Intermediate fasting & 5 2 diet

Intermediate or intermittent fasting is one of the main principles of this particular weight loss program, and as such, it is crucial to first clarify what this means to help you achieve your weight loss goals. Fasting is certainly not a new concept, in fact, individuals have been fasting for a long time and for different reasons.

The term fasting may leave some people intimidated, or even scared sometimes. However, when done correctly, fasting can certainly benefit people in many different ways and should not cause any harm. Individuals may decide to fast for many different reasons, and this rather radical process was once strictly linked with religious beliefs. Many years ago, Plato, Aristotle, and Socrates (Greek philosophers), believed that fasting was useful and had healing properties. Also, many fans of Yoga cleanse their body and mind by practicing fasting, as a natural way to cleanse their body.

In this century, fasting has been recommended for health benefits as well as weight loss. So, the 5 2 diet is following these recommendations. Many scientific studies have reported that fasting can actually be more efficient at times than surgery or medical procedures. The property of healing you get by fasting can be physical, emotionally and spiritually very powerful. Cleansing your body and letting it regenerate itself can be such as great way to improve your health. This book will help you understand how beneficial it can be, and certainly a great method to be able to shed the pounds you have accumulated over the years.

In the last 15 years or so, nutritionists and medical professionals, have come together to study and analyze the fasting process closely. Many personal trainers have also suggested that fasting can help in losing weight and have been promoting the benefits. What they all agree on is that fasting has to include a predetermined period. You can't fast all the time and you can't do it sporadically. It has to be somewhat consistent, so your body gets used to a certain cycle.

It makes complete sense that you will be able to lose weight through fasting, because during that period your body will utilize your fat as its primary source of energy instead of sugars. Also, fasting helps the insulin sensitivity in your body, meaning that you will start tolerating sugars or carbs better as you go along. This means that the sugars will be more effectively transported throughout your bloodstream. Also, when you are fasting, you are giving your gut (digestive system) a break. So your overall metabolism can actually become more efficient at digesting and burning fat once it starts working again normally, or once you start feeding your body more calories.

If you are normally hungry every 3 or 4 hours, you will start building a tolerance to hunger. This will also contribute to a permanent long term weight control. The hormones in your body will start to distinguish between the real hunger signals and the others, so you will start avoiding excessive eating patterns (binging).

We will find out more specifically what the benefits of fasting are in the next chapter are and how the 5 2 diet will help you lose the extra unwanted weight.

Chapter 2
Benefits associated with fasting

What interests us specifically with fasting, is primarily weight loss. Fasting is a safe way to lose excess pounds, and as long as it is well controlled and intermittent or intermediate as we have already discussed, your body will start burning the unwanted fat faster. Because you are giving your digestive system a break, your metabolism will work better and you can burn calories more rapidly than before. Nothing is "easy" per se, of course. Any diet or new way of eating and living requires conscious effort. What the 5 2 diet represents is a simple diet to follow while you don't have to purchase any specific products, supplements. You eat real food and healthy food. You simply have to control your portions and your caloric intake, on the 2 days you select as your fasting days.

The other reason why fasting will help you lose weight is because the hunger feelings of yours will change. No one has ever been truly starving after fasting for 3 or 4 hours. So, your body is not usually exposed to starvation. But when you trick it into fasting, it will change its ways of thinking and start experiencing true hunger. So, it is like reeducating your body to what the truth really is. After a while, when you eat smaller and less amounts of food, you will feel fuller faster than you used to, and will automatically lose weight from eating less.

On top of readjusting your body's feelings of hunger, you will change your eating habits for the better. It is the perfect time in your life to hit the reset button and teach your body what your new eating patterns will be. For example, if you decide not to eat anymore after 7 pm, make it a habit. Soon enough, you will get used to it and so will your body. Also, allow yourself to eat some foods you love, in moderation on the days you are not fasting.

As mentioned before, many philosophers used fasting to improve their body functions, including healing, and to also stimulate their thinking processes (brain function). It has been confirmed in fact that fasting boosts the production of a protein called brain-derived neurotrophic factor (BDNF). This protein triggers chemicals promoting cerebral health. More specifically, certain neurological diseases such as Parkinson's disease and Alzheimer's can be positively affected by fasting.

You don't need to practice yoga or meditation when you choose the 5 2 diet. However, when you fast, you could use that new eating experience to also reflect on other aspects of your life. By feeling lighter and more energized, you can have the energy to experience new things and feel better emotionally, spiritually and physically. So give it a try.

Your immune system will also benefit from intermittent fasting. When your body is fasting, the inflammation in your body is reduced. By reducing the amount of stress imposed on your body when it is actively working and digestion, it will be in better shape to fight off infections if needed. More energy and strength will be left to your body to battle anything that comes its way, including cancer if it occurs.

You will also be pleased with the way your skin will start looking healthier when you decide to fast. Your skin conditions can also be greatly improved by fasting and acne can also be prevented, as you are cleaning the toxins out of your liver and your kidneys. It's like doing a spring cleaning in your body.

Your level of blood sugar can be

impacted as well. Fasting can in fact have an impact on insulin sensitivity. So, if you tolerate carbs better, insulin will become more effective and the nutrients, including glucose, will be carried through your bloodstream more efficiently.

Finally, the long term effects of fasting are non-negligible. According to some studies, you can prolong your longevity if you practice fasting on a regular basis. The less you eat the less your body has to work to maintain its activities, the longer it will be able to perform its duties properly. Your metabolism will be slower as you are aging, so your digestive system will thank you when you give it less food to digest every day. Adopting the 5 2 diet long term is actually recommended is it works well for you, so you can fully enjoy the health benefits indefinitely.

Chapter 3
How does the 5 2 diet plan really works?

Alright, now let's get into the heart of the subject, and talk about how exactly the 5 2 diet works and what you should expect when you start following this program.

First, when following this program you will need to eat normally 5 days out of 7 and restrict your caloric intake to about 500 calories for women and 600 calories for men on the other 2 chosen fasting days. This caloric intake is significantly lower than a normal day as you can tell, and although it falls under intermittent fasting, you are still consuming minimal calories. On a non-fasting day, men should aim to consume about 2400 calories and women should eat around 2000 calories' worth of food.

You can select two consecutive or non-consecutive days, this is up to you. But try to select days that work well for you and that you can realistically fast and perform your regular activities normally. Some people like to spread them apart and choose to fast on Mondays and Thursdays, but you can also pick Tuesdays and Fridays. During the rest of the week, you should consume healthy and balanced meals. If you choose to eat unhealthy during the remaining 5 days, don't expect to lose weight. There is no miracle solution here. You will lose weight if you program your body correctly and feed it the right foods. Fasting can't compensate for your overeating on other days, so follow these simple rules and you will start losing some weight in no time.

Now remember we said that the 5 2 diet was also called the fast diet. Why is that? It is fast, because as soon as you start fasting, you will become more efficient at burning the accumulated fat instead of the calories you have been ingesting. Your metabolism will work better and faster and that's why you will be able to rapidly get thinner one pound at a time.

A normal period of fasting is usually defined as no eating for 36 hours. So for example, if you eat your diner around 7pm, on Wednesday night, you would not eat your next meal until Thursday morning around 7am. In the 5 2 diet, however, we suggest that instead of waiting 36 hours, you only wait 24 hours or less. So, you stop eating on Wednesday night at 7pm and you eat again around 1pm, or lunch time the next day. In this case, you would only have to fast for 17 hours. Again, you can adjust the fasting time to what works the best for you, depending on your schedule and activities.

Some people will wonder if fasting is bad for them, because they will be cutting so many calories from their diet. Not at all. Cutting back on your caloric intake twice a week won't harm you. Remember, our ancestors used to go long hours or days without eating, having to hunt for their food, and that was never a problem. Your situation will be very far from that extreme. I bet if you try to think about the last time you were starving, you would have to think long and hard. Our society in general overeats, and this causes increased risks of developing diseases in addition to being overweight. So by fasting and reducing the calories you ingest two times a week, rest assured that it will not impact you negatively, but just the opposite.

If you decide to follow this diet plan, you should realistically expect to lose about 1 pound a week if you are a women and a little more if you are a man. Of course, there are many factors that can influence your weight loss, but you should definitely avoid overeating or eating junk food on your "normal days" so you don't void the benefits of the fasting. Your total weight loss will vary from one individual to another. Some people will lose a few pounds, others a few dozen. Make sure you step on the scale before starting the 5 2 diet, so you know exactly where you are starting from, and after that, weighing yourself once a week should be sufficient. To be more accurate and also to celebrate your achievements, you should also take the time to measure your chest, waist and hips. Don't be surprised if your weight loss is greater at the beginning of the diet, as that is normal. If you follow the diet correctly, it can be very effective. The fact that you are fasting certainly promotes weight loss, but remember the fewer calories ingested during your non fasting days is what makes a big difference.

Studies have shown that some individuals who adopted this diet plan have lost up to 7% of their waist circumference or abdominal fat. It is known that belly fat can be very harmful to you, so this is a great benefit of the diet as well. The overall weight loss for many people who undertake this diet will be between 3% and 8% if they stick to the plan for about 24 weeks or so. Also, what is great to know is that the weight loss caused by fasting methods such as this one, will not be directly related to the loss of muscle mass. So, it seems like the perfect choice: fat loss, and stable muscle mass.

To measure your waist, make sure you stand straight up, with your feet shoulder width apart. Place the tape measure directly on your skin, and breathe normally while you are doing so. Don't compress the measuring tape into your body, as this will falsify the reading. You should place the tape halfway between your lowest rib and the top of your hipbone, approximately in line with your belly button, and remember to write your numbers down.

When you decide to undertake to the 5 2 diet approach, you should really think about calculating some body measurements so you can base your diet on facts. This will also give you another comparison point to be able to measure your progress and weight loss—other than the pounds lost when you weigh yourself.

First, the BMI or body mass index is based on your height and your weight and will give you an idea of your general body's composition. You can find BMI calculators online or predetermined charts that would make your task easier or divide your height in kilograms by your height in centimeters. The higher the number is, the more body fat someone has. A normal weight BMI should be anywhere between 18.5 and 24.9. So, if you exceed this reading, you know for sure you need to lose weight, especially body fat and the 5 2 diet will help you do so. Monitor your progress over the next weeks following the start of your diet.

Next, you should also look at your basal metabolic rate or BMR. This refers to the amount of calories you burn n a 24 hours period while doing absolutely nothing. Again, these aids can be looked up online, and you should do so to find yours. To obtain the BMR, you simply have to enter your weight and height.

Finally it can also be interesting to

calculate your TDEE, or total daily energy expenditure. In this way, you can understand what type of exercise and how much you should perform daily to reach your goal. Just like the BMR, you will use your weight and height, but you will also consider the amount of activities performed daily to better identify the real amount of calories you burn in a typical day. You will then have an idea of how many calories you burn, and how many more calories you technically should burn to lose weight.

Although the ultimate goal of this program is to lose weight, it's important to understand that you can also improve many other aspects of your health by following this diet. Hopefully you will shed the extra pounds of which you want to rid yourself, but the 5 2 diet can also have a very positive impact on your cholesterol levels. You can expect to bring your triglyceride levels down by about 20% in a 12 week period. Also during the same amount of time, your good cholesterol levels, or LDL should increase, and the levels of leptin can go down as much as 40%. The levels of CRP (C - reactive protein) will also be reduced, and any inflammation in your body will lessen. Make sure you check your cholesterol and blood sugar readings by visiting your doctor regularly. You can also measure your resting pulse, and that will be a great indicator of your overall health.

Because this diet is a natural one, simply by readjusting your calorie consumption you can certainly practice this plan for a long time if it works well for you. Even after losing the unwanted weight, you can keep applying the principles of the 5 2 diet. It can only work to benefit you long term, as you have already read in chapter 2.

Of course, no diet plan would be worth anything without incorporating some type of exercise routine. The 5 2 diet is no exception to the rule. Make sure you are physically active on a regular basis, just as you would be with any other diet or weight loss program.

Now, in the scenario where you are not losing the weight that you were hoping to lose, here are a few tips to follow.

You could actually switch the diet plan from 5 2 to a 4:3 plan. This means that instead of fasting 2 days a week, you would lower your calorie count 3 days a week and eat normally the other 4 days. For other individuals, it is better to use the 6:1 diet plan. This means that you can fast only one day, and eat normally 6 days out of the week. Perhaps you are a very active individual or you don't like fasting much. Either way, if you try the 6:1 diet and it works well, it could be a better solution for you. You could also opt for this solution if after a while being on the original 5 2 diet you reach a plateau and want to lose some additional pounds.

Remember, that losing weight is great. However, the overall goal is to lose fat and be healthier. You should also make sure you closely monitor the other indicators as mentioned earlier, and not only your scale.

If you are losing a lot of circumference around your waist, then you know you are doing something right.

If you are not satisfied with the weight you are shedding, think about changing your physical activities, and just make yourself get out and move more. Instead of going to the gym twice a week, go 4 times a week or add a few walks around the neighborhood.

Cut the calories you drink if cutting the calories you eat does not seem to be doing the trick. Avoid all sugary drinks, coffees, teas, alcohol and concentrate on drinking more water.

Finally, just like you would with any other diet, you could keep a journal. This helps many people be even more conscious of what they eat, drink and the physical activities they perform daily. At first, pay attention to the calories contained in each slice of bread, portion of meat, or piece of fruit. Soon, it will be second nature, and you will know approximately how to correctly add up your calories for the day. By writing down everything you eat, you will definitely think twice at times before snacking on unhealthy food or eating a second portion.

Chapter 4
Example of meal plan for 5 2 diet beginners

Are you ready? Let's do this! Let's establish a meal plan that will allow you to lose the weight you have been wanting to get rid of for a long time. If you are consistent and put in the required effort, this 5 2 diet will not fail you.

On fasting days

You will find below a list of suggested food to eat on fasting days. You will eventually be able to create your own meal plans as you figure out what foods can be substituted for other less diet friendly foods, and you can actually get more creative as you go along. You can also write down th e recipes or foods you enjoyed the most in a journal, so that you can remember to prepare them again or buy the required ingredients on your next trip to the grocery store.

Remember, on the fasting days, you will restrict your caloric intake to 500-600 calories, so make sure you pay attention to the food labels and if you are not certain, you can always use the internet to research the number of calories associated with certain food items.

The foods below are only suggestions. You can actually eat pretty much what you like, as long as you keep your daily caloric intake under the suggested amount.

- Avoid any processed foods (frozen dinners, deli meats), and favor natural and fresh ingredients (so you know exactly what you are eating).

- Obviously avoid any junk foods such as cookies, donuts, French fries etc.

- Favor foods that are filling but low in calories.

- The foods you select should ideally be high in proteins and fibers.

- If you consume dairy products, make sure they are low fat.

- Drink plenty of water. Remember you can't really drink too much water, aim for 8 glasses per day.

- Other than water, you can drink black coffee and unsweetened tea. If you do add milk in your beverages, make sure to count the calories. Although diet drinks and diet sodas are low in calories, remember to consume them in moderation because the artificial sweeteners can still throw off your blood sugar and are very unhealthy for you.

- Eat small portions of lean meats, to get your protein intakes. Also, eat eggs, but favor hardboiled eggs and poached eggs over fried ones. Also, bake or grill your meat to avoid additional unhealthy fats. Eat fish as well. Soy is a great source of protein too, so try eating tofu.

- Eat plenty of vegetables. It is recommended to eat the green leafy ones such as spinach, and kale. Avoid the starchy vegetables, such as potatoes, on your fasting days as they contain a lot more calories.

- Soups can certainly fill you up and if prepare them correctly can contain a lot of nutrients. Look into bone broths or vegetables soups.

- You can also prepare delicious salads with multiple vegetables, just make sure you use low fat dressings, or even better simply drizzles of olive oil and balsamic vinegar.

- Most fruits contain a lot of sugar that could send your caloric intake to the roof quickly. If you are going to eat fruits during your fasting days, favor berries (blueberries, raspberries, strawberries, blackberries).

- When you feel the need to snack on fast days, chose carefully. Eat a handful of nuts, such as almonds or walnuts. Snack on celery sticks or a few slices of apple.

- You probably want to avoid alcohol all together during your fasting days. If you include a glass of wine or a beer, you have to calculate that 150-250 calories into your total for the day, so it does not leave many calories for the rest of your food.

- Finally, keep the carbohydrates (carbs) to a minimum during these 2 chosen days. Don't eat white bread, pasta or rice. It is actually a good habit to eliminate these foods all together even during your non fasting days and replace them with whole grains such as oats, quinoa, wheat, and brown rice. But remember that if you eat a portion of carbs, even the healthy ones, you will have to calculate these calories towards your 500-600 calorie goal.

You can choose how you allocate the foods and calories. Some people like to eat a large breakfast and 2 very light meals the rest of the day. Some people prefer to eat 2 larger meals. Remember the caloric intake is only 500 or 600 calories, so you have to make sure you don't go over, as that's really what matters during these 2 fasting days.

It is a good idea to evaluate the type of activities you have planned on these fasting days and eating accordingly. If you have a lot of meetings back to back at work, you might benefit from eating a powerful breakfast and lighter lunch and supper. There is no one-size-fits-all solution, because we all have our own preferences. If you are already in the habit of skipping breakfast, you might as well continue skipping it and concentre your caloric intake on other meals. There is going to be a period of trial and error and you will be able to find what works bests you. If you like to have a traditional meal on your plate, simply make sure your portions are a lot smaller (a few ounces of tuna, salad, and cottage cheese for example).

Here are some examples:

Snacks

- ✓ A handful of almonds
- ✓ An avocado or a banana
- ✓ ½ cup of low fat plain yoghurt
- ✓ Nutty energy bar (see recipe chapter 5)
- ✓ Slice of apple with 1 tbsp. of almond butter
- ✓ 1 Cup of edamame with salt
- ✓ 1 cup of popcorn (no butter)
- ✓ ½ cup of pumpkin seeds

Breakfast

- ✓ Spinach omelette (*see recipe chapter 5*)

- ✓ ½ cup oatmeal and blackberries

- ✓ Tomato slices with balsamic vinegar and hardboiled egg

- ✓ 1 cup of low fat low sodium baked beans with 1 slice of wheat bread

- ✓ Low calories watermelon smoothie (see recipe chapter 5)

Lunch

- ✓ Low calorie tomato soup or miso soup (*see recipe chapter 5*)

- ✓ Grilled chicken (a few ounces) and ½ cup of cooked asparagus

- ✓ Zucchini noodles cooked in olive oil with crumbled feta cheese

- ✓ Asian Salad (*see recipe chapter 5*)

- ✓ Pita bread with 2 tbsp. of hummus

- ✓ Sardine' salad (see recipe chapter 5)

Dinner

- ✓ Few ounces of baked salmon and steamed broccoli

- ✓ Half green bell pepper stuffed with low fat ricotta cheese and other veggies

- ✓ Green bean's delight (*see recipe chapter 5*)

- ✓ Sautéed tofu and brown rice

- ✓ Shirataki Noodles & shrimp (*see recipe chapter 5*)

- ✓ Grilled vegetable's kebab (with zucchinis, eggplant, tomatoes mushrooms) with cottage cheese

Chapter 5
A few 5:2 diet friendly recipes

Nutty Energy bar

1 Serving = 1 square 135 calories

Recipe serves 16

Ingredients

- ✓ 1/3 cup dark chocolate chips
- ✓ 1/3 unsalted peanuts
- ✓ 1 ½ cup oats
- ✓ ¼ cup unsalted butter
- ✓ ¼ light brown sugar

- ✓ ¼ quality olive oil

- ✓ 2 tbsp. rice malt syrup

- ✓ Zest and juice of 1 lemon

Preparation

Preheat oven to 350 degrees F. Spray a square baking pan with non-stick olive oil.

In a bowl mix the peanuts, oats and lemon zest.

Next, in a small skillet combine olive oil, butter, brown sugar, lemon juice and rice malt syrup. Heat on low and mix well until everything is smooth and melted.

Next, pour this mixture on top of the peanut mixture. Stir well so all the mixture is coated. Transfer the mix into the baking pan and press firmly.

Bake in the oven for 20 to 25 minutes.

Finally, right after removing from the oven, place the chocolate chips on top and let them melt.

Once it cools down, cut them into 16 squares.

Spinach omelette

Recipe serves 1

1 serving =1 medium egg and 1 cup of fresh spinach = 95 calories

Ingredients

- ✓ 1 egg
- ✓ 1 cup fresh spinach
- ✓ Salt and pepper
- ✓ Fresh herbs of your choice (oregano, cilantro)

Preparation

It is as simple as it sounds, simply spray a pan with non-stick oil or use some olive oil. Cook the spinach for a few minutes. Crack the egg in a bowl and whisk it. Add the beaten egg and the seasonings.

Watermelon Smoothie

Serving = 1 glass = 155 calories

Recipe serves 2

Ingredients

- ✓ 2 cups of watermelon
- ✓ 1 cup of raspberries
- ✓ 1 cup of low fat Greek yoghurt
- ✓ Ice

Preparation

Simply blend all the ingredients well together.

Miso soup

Serving = 1 cup = 100 calories

Recipe serves 2

Ingredients

- ✓ 2 small Japanese miso paste sachets (your favorite brand)
- ✓ 1 clove garlic - crushed
- ✓ ½ tsp grated fresh ginger
- ✓ ½ cup of sliced mushrooms
- ✓ ½ chopped sweet onion
- ✓ Olive oil
- ✓ Dash soy sauce
- ✓ Boiling water (2 ½ cups)

Preparation

Pour 2 ½ cups of boiling water into a pot and mix in the miso paste until completely dissolved.

Cook the onion in olive oil in a skillet. Then mix in all ingredients (mushrooms, onions, cabbage, soya sauce, garlic and ginger). Let the soup simmer for about 15 minutes.

You could add some chicken breast cubes if you like, and simply count the additional calories.

Sardine's salad

Serving = 1 cup = 170 calories

Recipe serves 4

Ingredients

- ✓ mixed greens
- ✓ 1 small chopped
- ✓ ½ small chopped red onion
- ✓ 2 tsp. capers
- ✓ 2 cans sardines (skinless and in oil)
- ✓ handful black olives or green olives (your favorite)
- ✓ 1 tbsp. balsamic vinegar

Preparation

Lay the mixed greens on your pate and then sprinkle some olives, red onions, tomatoes and capers.

Then cut up the sardines and place them on your bed of greens, drizzle with balsamic vinegar.

Asian salad

Recipe serves 2

1 serving: 130 calories

Ingredients

- ✓ 1 small cooked boneless and skinless chicken breast, cut into small pieces
- ✓ 2 cups of mixed greens of your choice (the darker the better)
- ✓ ¼ cup chopped cucumber
- ✓ 1 chopped green onion

Dressing

- ✓ 1 tbsp. honey
- ✓ Salt and pepper

- ✓ 1 tsp. coriander (or chopped fresh herbs if you can)
- ✓ 1 tbsp. fish sauce of your choice
- ✓ Zest and juice of 1 lime

Preparation

Prepare the dressing by mixing together the lime zest, juice, fish sauce, and honey and seasonings.

Then place the mixed greens on the plate, the chicken breast, the cucumber and green onion. Drizzle with the dressing and enjoy.

Green bean's delight

Serving = 1 cup = 145 calories

Recipe serves 4

Ingredients

- ✓ 2 red bell peppers
- ✓ 2 yellow bell peppers
- ✓ ½ chopped red onion
- ✓ 2 cups green beans
- ✓ 2 cup of mixed greens

Dressing

- ✓ 6 tbsp. olive oil
- ✓ 2 tbsp. balsamic vinegar
- ✓ 1 tsp honey

✓ 1 tbsp. freshly grated ginger

Preparation

Preheat the oven to 400°F

Place the peppers, cut-side down, on a baking sheet and cook them for about 30 minutes. Afterwards, let them cool down. Peel the pepper's skins and chop them.

Then, cook the green beans in boiling water for about 5 minutes, don't let them get soggy. Drain, and place them with the peppers in a large bowl.

Finally, prepare the dressing. Mix all the ingredients listed for the dressing in a separate bowl.

Serve room temperature, by pouring the dressing on your vegetables.

Shirataki (or vermicelli rice noodles) Noodles & Shrimp

Serving = 1 cup = 210 calories

Recipe serves 1

Ingredients

- ✓ 2 cups Shirataki Noodles
- ✓ 1 cup medium shrimp
- ✓ 2 chopped green onions
- ✓ 1 minced clove garlic
- ✓ 1 tbsp. minced ginger
- ✓ ½ cup of snow peas
- ✓ ½ cup Chinese cabbage or leafs
- ✓ 1 tbsp. olive oil or sesame oil
- ✓ 2 tsp. of soy sauce (low fat low, sodium)

✓ 2 tbsp. lemon juice

✓ 1 tbsp., cayenne pepper

✓ salt

Preparation

First step is to prepare the noodles as instructed on the package or the box.

Then, heat the olive oil in a large skillet and cook the onions, ginger and garlic for a few minutes.

Add the shrimp and cook until pink.

Add the remaining vegetables (snow peas, cabbage), including the cayenne pepper and cook for about another 7-8 minutes.

Add the soy sauce, lemon juice and

bring to a boil. Season with salt if you judge necessary.

Serve the dish on a bed of Shirataki noodles.

Chapter 6
FAQ's

Can anyone follow the 5 2 diet?

Children under 18 as well as pregnant women should not adopt this diet plan. If you are trying to conceive or have issues with fertility, it is not a good idea to be on any diet actually. If you have been diagnosed or have self-diagnosed eating disorders, then the 5 2 diet is not for you. Evidently, if you are underweight, you should not be wanting to lose weight nor start the 5 2 diet.

Also, if you are feeling sick or are running fever, you should not start this diet, you should wait until you recover completely. If you are suffering from diabetes type 1, or taking diabetic medications, please do not start the 5 2 diet and consult your primary care doctor for additional explanations. Actually, if you have any chronic medical conditions or are taking any medications on a regular basis you should always speak with your doctor first.

Additionally, if you have recently had surgery, wait until you are completely well again, up to 6 to 8 weeks after surgery, to start this diet plan. Finally, it is not recommend for elderly individuals to try this intermittent fasting plan, as their health might be already fragile and this could do more harm than good.

Are there side effects associated with this diet?

Like with any other diet plan, you can certainly experience hunger, especially during the first week or so. However, no major side effects are expected. There may possibly be some trouble sleeping, if you are feeling hungry during the fasting days. You could also experience constipation at times, but you should remember to drink plenty of water to avoid this discomfort. Also, some individuals will have headaches. The typical symptoms you feel when you first start dieting. Nothing more, nothing less. You should not feel shaky or terribly weak. Your body will adjust and is actually work to preserve your blood sugar at a certain level so you can go without food for several hours.

Will I be constantly hungry and irritable during the fasting periods?

At first, it will be normal to feel hunger, and your body will have to get used to it, however, it should not be extreme. After just a few days, most people who have tried the diet say that it becomes much easier. You will eventually start feeling energized when you are fasting, as you will feel lighter and will be able to give your body a break from working as hard as it does. As far as irritable, you should not be any more moody than with any other diet or lifestyle change you would try. It takes a little while to get adjusted, but then it becomes routine. So, if you are feeling hungry, try to occupy or distract yourself. Go for a car ride, a walk, or have a tall glass of water or low calorie drink—water works great.

If you are still not feeling well several days in, you have to be in tune with your body. Make sure you don't drastically change all your habits. If you have never tried to fast before, for example, it's a good idea to keep healthy snacks close by in case you start feeling really week or tired. If you are feeling ill, you want to stop the diet and/or consult with a health professional. Fasting might not be the right solution for everyone, so just make sure you listen to the signs your body is giving you. Also, if you are a woman for example, you might wait to start until your menstrual cycle is over, or that you don't have too many activities to attend with the children to start.

Remember, you will not create a starvation mode for your body, you are only lowering your caloric intake for a few days, so it is not a dramatic change. It is enough of a change to make a difference and help you lose weight, but not a survival status for you.

Should I exercise anyway while I am fasting?

You certainly should be able to maintain your regular activities: work, errands, cooking, cleaning. You should even be able to take walks, go for a swim or a bike ride without problems. However, it is probably a good idea to avoid very intense physical activities. Especially until you truly understand what fasting does to your body and that you get used physically to this calories withdraw.

If you do choose to exercise, remember that you should not compensate and eat over the 500 or 600 calories max for the day.

That's not the goal. If you decide to exercise, then welcome the additional burned calories and hopefully the extra pounds lost for that week. Make sure you monitor how you feel during a workout and if you are not feeling well, always slow down or stop immediately what you are doing.

Now of course, exercising is certainly recommend during the week to maintain an overall healthy lifestyle and loose the weight faster. Not only can you shed the pounds, but you will contribute to a healthier you by helping your body in fighting many diseases. Incorporate fitness in your life whenever you can. Taking the stairs at work, parking your car farther at the mall, and going to the convenience store by walking will make you add many steps to your day and burn many additional calories.

How can I make sure I do not regain weight?

Often diet plans help you lose a significant amount of weight at first and then unfortunately 6 month or less than year later, you have gained all the weight back. In some cases, individuals even gain more weight back than they lost to begin with. How can you avoid that?

The 5 2 diet is particularly effective as a long term plan, because you are reprogramming your body to digest the food and perform other bodily functions better and faster. So, as long as you keep up with an overall healthy diet, you should be able to keep that weight off. As we have already said, you could continue with the fasting part time, a day or two a week if you like. But even if you choose not to do so, you can keep the pounds off your body if you don't go back to your old unhealthy eating habits. Keep the amount of proteins, healthy fats, and fibers high in your diet. This means you should include lean chicken, pork, tofu, eggs, turkey, along with lots of vegetables and whole grain cereals. Favor coconut oil and olive oil for cooking, and avoid any fried foods.

Finally, because you will be in touch with your body better than ever, you can tell right away if you are starting to feel uncomfortable or tight in your clothes. If that becomes the case, don't wait until you have gained all the weight back, but act on it right way instead. Go back to a few days of fasting or review your new eating habits to make sure you are complying. Don't forget to also evaluate how much exercise you incorporate into your life and that will make a big difference as well.

Conclusion

If you want to lose weight, it's not rocket science, brain surgery, or even a big secret—you have to change your eating habits. As you have learned in this book, changing what you eat is sometimes not enough, but changing when you eat it and the portions is what will work better and faster for you. The 5 2 diet is an intermittent fasting plan that allows you to maintain your regular activities by controlling your caloric intake. Two days a week you will follow the guidelines explained in the book and significantly lower the calories you ingest.

In this way you will teach your body to burn the fat your body would normally be storing in your reserves, and by consequence, lose the pounds you want to lose. Follow some of the proposed recipes in this book and meal's suggestions. Make sure that on fasting days you do not eat more than 500 or 600 calories total. Favor some natural foods, vegetables, healthy fats, proteins and low fat dairy products. Do not fry your food, but instead grill or bake your meat and fish. Get creative, you can do it even with low caloric intake meals, so you don't get bored and you do get enough nutrients to keep doing all your daily activities. If you are looking for quick fillers, soups, teas, or salads will satisfied you and will allow you to respect this diet 5 2 principles on the designated fasting days.

We have also mentioned to you the many other health benefits you can enjoy when you practice fasting, even if it is intermittent fasting. You can greatly reduce many other risks of certain diseases, which is priceless. You will feel better physically and mentally and your life overall will be better. There is no reason why you should be worried about fasting. It has been practiced for a long time and this diet plan is very gentle. You can also learn to modify your diet as you go, once you have reached your weight loss goals. That way, without going back to your old bad eating habits, you can create your own routine.

However, remember that you should closely monitor how you feel and how your body reacts to these changes you are making. You should not feel excessively tired or lethargic. Yes, you will be hungry at first perhaps, and this is normal. But soon your body will adjust and get used to this lower caloric intake. If you are genuinely concerned about the way you feel, you should consult with your regular health professional. Otherwise, you will be surprised at how efficient and fast this 5 2 diet shows results. That's right, in just about a month, more or less, you will already have lost weight and will be well on your way to a heathier and skinner you.

It's important to remember that what we eat plays a major role in our heath and weight. But, exercising is also a key element to a healthy lifestyle. Don't forget to be active, and you will not only be able to shed some pounds faster, but will also prevent many diseases and keep your heart healthy. If it works better for you, you can skip intense workouts during the two fasting das and concentrate on walking or other normal activities. The rest of the week you should adopt a regular exercise routine and stick with it.

Everyone is looking for a miracle solution. The bad news is, this does not exist. The good news is that the 5 2 diet is a great solution to your weight problem. You don't need any special equipment or special foods to start this diet, only a lot of motivation and self-control at first, and soon enough, your body will have resigned itself to this new eating program. The 5 2 diet will help you save money as well! Good luck and remember that fasting does not have to be scary.

Thank you again for reading this book!

I hope this book was able to help you realize how healthy fasting with the diet 5 2 can be for you if done the right way.

Finally, if you enjoyed this book, then I'd like to ask you for a favor, would you be kind enough to leave a review for this book on Amazon? It'd be greatly appreciated!

Thank you and good luck!

Made in the USA
Coppell, TX
01 March 2020

16365510R00046